I0426627

The New You

Tips and Tricks to Losing Weight, Get in Shape Safely and Keeping It Off

Daniel Michael

Copyright

© 2012 by Daniel Michael

ISBN: 978-1-304-71468-8

All rights reserved. The reproduction or utilization of this work in whole in part, in any form by any print, electronic, mechanical or other means, now known or hereafter invented, including xerography, photocopying and recording, or in any information storage or retrieval system is forbidden without the written permission of the publisher.

Please do not participate in or encourage piracy of any copyrighted materials in any form. To do so is a violation of the author's rights.

Terms of Use

Any information provided in this book is through the author's interpretation. The author has done strenuous work to reassure the accuracy of this subject. If you wish you attempt any of the practices provided in this book, you are doing so with your own responsibility. The author will not be held accountable for any misinterpretations or misrepresentations of the information provided here.

All information provided is done so with every effort to represent the subject, but does not guarantee that your life will change. The author shall not be held liable for any direct or indirect damages that result from reading this book.

Contents

Introduction

No matter if you are a few pounds overweight, or several, if you have picked up this book, it is because you are ready to get serious about losing the weight and to maintain a healthy weight.

Our society has conditioned us to feel that large is bad, and skinny is good.

We are bombarded with advertisements with skinny models, numerous fat loss pills, meal plans, fad diets and gyms, all promising the perfect body for you.

Most of us who lose weight, do so because we want to be healthy, we are trying to be healthy for us, not to fit in.

Fad diets promise quick results, but even if they deliver, the results are often on short-term and can actually be damaging to your body.

You will never lose weight by diet alone, and you will never be healthy with exercise alone.

This book is your guide on how to change your eating habits so that you start losing weight quickly, and how to lose it even faster through exercise.

Losing weight involves changes in not only what you eat, but also how you eat.

You do not have to subscribe to fancy meal plan services, or spend hours cooking complicated meals.

Learn to eat, feel full, and feel energized, all while losing weight.

Likewise, it is possible to get fit and healthy without an expensive gym membership, and you will be surprised at how you can fit enough exercise into your already busy schedule to help you boost your weight loss.

With diet and exercise, you will get results.

Several fad diets, and indeed, even some reality TV shows have people losing well over 5-10 pounds a week.

Doctors recommend only 1-2 pounds a week; some of the dangers of rapid weight loss:

Rapid weight loss can contribute to the likelihood of developing an eating disorder.

Increased risk of having heart problems, including going into cardiac arrest.

Increased chance of developing depression or anxiety disorders

Increased risk of developing kidney stones or having your kidneys fail.

We will help you shed your pounds in a healthy way, and in such a way that you will not feel hungry, starved, or underfed.

You will actually be eating healthy, which will make you feel energized, and healthier.

Our simple, yet effective exercise plan will allow you to add that one-two punch to your weight loss and keep you fit and trim.

You must be ready to make these changes and commit to them over the long term.

We know this is not easy, which is why we recommend that you make the changes to your diet slowly, by setting them as goals, which we go over in our goal setting section.

It is a lot easier to transition to a healthier lifestyle when you can do it in steps and stages instead of all at once, which can make you feel overwhelmed.

By setting smaller goals, all leading up to the main long-term goal, you will be more motivated to continue as you reach each goal, and motivation is a big factor.

You have to want to make these changes in order for them to stick.

Same with your exercise, you should be very careful to not overdo your fitness routine, especially if you are out of shape, or not used to exercising, the goal is to get in shape safely, and to keep it off.

Biting off more than you can chew will only discourage you and could have negative health consequences.

You should also be aware of any big life changes that have either just happened, or are about to happen, because things like that are stressful enough on their own, trying to change your eating habits can just add more stress.

Same with if you are having emotional problems, or going through times with lots of stress, that can trigger emotional eating; you might want to get a handle on any underlying stressors that trigger emotional eating on your part.

Debunking Diet Myths

To begin with, we will go over several popular diet myths, and yes, they are myths.

We will explain all of the popular myths so that you know why they are not true. Some of these will surprise you.

You gain weight if you eat late at night

False, it does not matter when you eat, it matters how many calories you have had throughout the entire day. Timing has nothing to do with it.

If I only eat salad for lunch, I will lose weight faster

Not true because, lettuce by itself does not have a high nutritional value, and it will not stay with you long.

To feel satisfied when eating salads, make sure that your salad has some lean protein with it, such as turkey or chicken and even some cheese.

This will keep you from getting hungry shortly after eating.

If I skip a meal, I will lose weight faster

The idea here is that if you skip a meal, you will take in fewer calories, therefore will lose weight faster.

The problem with skipping a meal is, that when your body needs food and does not have it, your metabolism will slow down to respond to this "starvation;" which is exactly how your body sees a skipped meal.

A slower metabolism means that you will be processing food slower, slowing down your weight loss, which is the opposite of what you are trying to achieve.

When you skip a meal, you will also tend to overeat at your next meal, which also defeats the point.

Instead of skipping meals, make them healthier meals.

Low-carb diets work!

In a way this is true; but not in the way that you think.

Low-carb diets will not provide your body with the amount of carbohydrates that it requires daily.

In response, your body will begin to burn its stored carbohydrates for energy, which releases water.

The rapid weight loss that you will experience from a low-carb diet is simply water weight.

Another problem with the low-carb diet is that the foods marketed as low-carb, while being low-carb are often very high in calories.

If it says sugar free or fat free, it is diet friendly

Just because something says it is fat free or sugar free, does not mean it is good for you.

In order to taste good, these foods are often full of artificial ingredients and Trans fats that we just are not meant to eat large quantities of.

Food manufactures want consumers to think that they are eating health foods; when in fact, they are not.

Pay attention to the label, and the calorie count. Eat these items in moderation, and you will be fine.

I have to give up my favorite foods in order to lose weight

False, by depriving yourself of all of the things that you enjoy, you will only end up binge eating.

Having some of your favorite foods in moderation is perfectly acceptable, it will help curb your cravings and keep you motivated to stay on track.

Just remember to try to keep your calories in check, so instead of three or four cookies, have just one, and not every day.

Carbohydrates pack on the pounds

The reality of eating is that extra calories will make you gain weight, no matter what form you consume the calories in. If you cut out carbohydrates, you end up cutting out vegetables, fruits, and whole grains from your diet, all of which are essential to a well-balanced diet.

Limit your heavy carb foods, like pasta, instead of cutting out all carbs from your diet plan.

Setting Your Weight Loss Goals

The best way to achieve and maintain your weight loss is to break it out into goals.

If you are significantly overweight, you should probably see a doctor first, to make sure that your health is okay, and to keep your blood pressure monitored.

Several websites online will help you set your goals and track your progress.

You can download apps that will help you count calories as well as set how many calories you should eat daily, myfitnesspal.com is only one such tool, there are many other free tools at your disposal.

Have you heard of a SMART goal? No? SMART stands for:

Specific

Measurable

Attainable

Realistic

Timely

Have a weight loss journal or chart and set your goals up in sections. Set your long-term goal or your ultimate target weight and then set up smaller goals for reaching that goal.

For example, if you want to lose a total of 30 pounds, then set your goals up similar to this:

To have lost 6 pounds after 30 days

To have lost 12 pounds after 60 days

To have lost 18 pounds after 90 days

To have lost 24 pounds after 120 days

To have lost 30 pounds after 150 days

You should measure your progress weekly, and keep track of the results, either using an online tool, or in a written journal.

The best way to do this is to weigh yourself at the start of each week, and again at the end.

You can also set fitness goals, such as how many days a week to exercise, and for how long.

Track this using a fitness app, or in your journal as well.

Your goals can also include your eating habits, such as make a goal to swap out one soda a day for a glass of water for the first week, make a goal of swapping out high sugar cereal with a bowl of oatmeal, make a goal of cutting back on your coffee by one cup, etc.

Make sure that your goals are attainable.

Do not set goals that are un-realistic, such as trying for at least 4+ pounds per week, or excess exercise.

Goals that push your body to the limit will do more damage than good.

You can also become depressed and want to give up if you set goals that you cannot meet.

Instead of turning your diet upside down all at once, incorporate your new healthy eating habits into your diet slowly and make some of those changes as your goals; small changes to your eating habits are a lot easier to deal with, and will be less likely to overwhelm you with a lot of changes in a short period of time.

Some examples are:

Add one serving of fresh fruit to your daily intake

Replace your whole milk with low-fat or non-fat milk

Replace one red meat meal with a leaner meat option

Extend your goals, or broaden them as you turn your beginning goals into intermediate goals.

For example, if to start with you decide that you will take a thirty minute walk every day, your next goal could be that after two weeks you increase it to forty-five minutes, and then after three weeks, a full hour.

The timing part means that you have a definite date to start with your fitness and you do not waiver from that.

Do not put the diet off for another week, set a date, and start it now.

Stay on top of your short-term and long-term goals.

Focus on the smaller goals, such as replace this food for that food, or loose x pounds in 30 days, instead of your long-term goal of ultimately weighing x pounds.

Understand that you might need to change your goals along the way, be flexible in your goals.

Remember, setbacks will happen, there will be weeks when you do everything right, but you are not losing weight.

Just never give up, and if you have to evaluate your food choices and replace one food for another in order to reach your goal, do so.

Remember, this is a long-term plan, designed to not only shed the weight but to help you keep it off.

Track your progress and celebrate each goal that you reach.

Reward yourself with a treat, see a movie, and buy a new piece of clothing.

You will have worked hard to reach each goal and you deserve to be rewarded for it.

Foods to Take Out of Your Diet

You already know that you need to change your diet, because what you have been eating, obviously is not working to help you lose weight.

This section will explain to you the foods that should be eaten in moderation, three times a week or less, and in limited amounts, or take out of your diet completely.

Alcohol

Alcohol is extremely high in calories; even the light versions of alcoholic beverages carry a very high calorie count.

If you are trying to cut back on calories, just by cutting back on the quantity of the alcohol that you drink, you will begin to cut your calorie intake greatly.

Not only is it high in calories, but because it actually a poison to our system, our liver has to kick in gear to process and detoxify the alcohol right away, which means other foods do not get processed quickly, such as fat.

Processed meats

Meats such as sausage, bacon, hot dogs, smoked meats, and lunchmeats are full of fillers, high in sodium and full of nitrates, which are used to preserve the meat. Sodium contributes to heart disease, nitrates have been linked to cancer, and fillers are all artificial ingredients that just make our system work harder to digest.

This goes for canned meat as well, the exception is that salmon, tuna, crab, sardines, mackerels, and anchovies are okay to keep in your diet, but be careful with how much you eat; they are still high in sodium, even though they have no fillers and nitrates.

Fruit drinks

Read the label carefully when shopping for juice or fruit drinks because the majority of what is on the shelves will be less than 10% fruit juice, they use high fructose corn syrup or other sugars to sweeten them and will have artificial flavors.

Find organic juice, or buy the fruit and juice it yourself.

Margarine, Vegetable Oil, and Shortening

These are high in Trans fats, which are the bad kind of fat.

You may think you are being health conscious by cooking with these, but you are not.

Trans fats will cause you to gain weight quicker and can lead to inflamed joints and make it so that you are more apt to develop heart disease or even cancer.

Butter is actually a better choice than using any of the above. You can also use extra virgin olive oil, or coconut oil to cook with.

Frozen dinners

Our world is fast paced, and the freezer section of any grocery store is full of frozen lunch and dinner choices, many that appear to have diet friendly names.

How surprised would you be to find out that these self-proclaimed healthy foods are not healthy at all?

Sure, they may be low enough in calories to look like a good diet food choice, but resist adding these to your cart.

These frozen meals are full of processed foods, artificial ingredients and have sky-high sodium levels.

The idea of being healthy is to put healthy food into your body, chemicals and artificial ingredients are not healthy.

Sodium can actually make you feel hungry, so even though you just ate, you will still feel hungry.

Aside from the above, and the usual bland taste of the food, the portions are small and chances are; will not fully satisfy your hungry, making you prone to snacking.

By eating these, you not only are filling your body with unhealthy ingredients but you will most likely end up overeating at the end of the day.

Fried Foods

You knew this was coming, and we bet you did not want to hear it, but there it is.

Frying adds Trans fats and/or saturated fats to the food that gets fried and packs a big calorie wallop as well.

Fried foods, especially fast food fried foods, are also full of preservatives and fillers as well.

Things like French fries and potato chips are also high in sodium and the artificial ingredients that they contain can be cancer-causing agents, on top of the high calorie and fat content.

Donuts are also in this group, full of sugar and fats, and a giant calorie count.

Other foods to watch out in this category are hash browns, tater tots, onion rings, and fried zucchini.

Soda

Soda is very high in calories, and if eating out, usually served in a giant cup, with an already calorie high meal.

In addition to calories, soda should be avoided for two other reasons; two of the main ingredients are high fructose corn syrup and phosphoric acid.

High fructose corn syrup is basically sugar in liquid form and allows us to intake more sugar at a time; this can contribute greatly to diabetes, obesity, high blood pressure, high cholesterol, tooth decay, and weight gain.

Phosphoric acid can contribute to osteoporosis because phosphoric acid not only interferes with digestion but it removed minerals from out of your bones.

Diet soda

Bet you thought you were safe by drinking diet soda, but you would be wrong. Not only are diet sodas bad for you because of the phosphoric acid, but they are loaded with artificial sweeteners.

Artificial sweeteners have been shown to trigger cravings, making you feel hungrier after eating something that contains them.

The most widely uses artificial sweetener is aspartame, which is known to have a series of bad effects to our health; such as diabetes, cancer, birth defects, alters our brain chemistry to the point that emotional disorders manifest.

Ice cream

We all love ice cream, but it is full of calories, sugar and fat and many brands use artificial flavors and other ingredients.

When eating ice cream, eat in moderation, and look for the brands that use real flavors as opposed to artificial, and you can curb your sweet tooth, without adding a bunch of unnatural ingredients into your body.

White Bread, pasta

When you eat bread and pasta, your body treats it like you are eating refined white sugar, which is empty calorie food.

Bread is not the enemy to the diet; white bread is, because of the white flour.

Foods You Should Be Eating

Oatmeal

We mean old-fashioned oatmeal, not the instant variety. Although tasty, the flavors in the instant kind are often artificial and not good for your health.

Although oatmeal is a carb, it is of the kind that releases slowly, which is beneficial when trying to reduce body fat.

Oatmeal is rich in protein, carbs and the good kind of fat; it also have nutrients such as vitamin E, zinc and iron, all of which help reduce cholesterol level.

So skip your sugar breakfast cereals and have a bowl of oatmeal instead, it will fill you up and give you the energy needed to start your day, without that sugar crash that cereal provide you with.

Whole wheat/whole grain products

A much healthier choice that white breads and enriched bread products because these bread products are low in calories, a good source of protein and contain vitamins and minerals that we need to be healthy.

Check your labels to make sure that the ingredients say whole wheat and not just wheat.

Meats

Avoid the processed meats, or smoked and processed meat products. Try to limit your red meat to three times a week, and make sure that when you eat red meat, that it is lean red meat.

Avoid cuts like prime rib, which are cuts of meat that are usually very fatty; instead opt for top round steak or flank steak.

Proteins are an important part of any diet plan because they are harder to digest, so your body actually works harder to digest proteins, helping to burn more calories.

Proteins also help you build muscle and improve your immune system. Some good meat choices are:

Chicken breasts / turkey breast

Shrimp

Cod

Rainbow trout

Lean ground sirloin

Ground turkey (use this in your ground beef recipes to replace the ground beef)

Buffalo – yes, ground buffalo is a healthy red meat

Salmon and tuna– wild caught is the best. These fish are high in Omega-3 fatty acids, which are good for you.

Eggs/egg whites

Eggs are an excellent source of protein and good way to kick start your day.

Eggs will help you feel full longer, and because of that, you will tend to snack less if you start your day off with a few eggs.

Add some cheese and some veggies to make a delicious omelet. It used to be thought that eggs would raise cholesterol, but that has been proven wrong.

Egg protein is the best protein to eat when trying to build muscle.

Green vegetables/vegetables

Popeye knew the secret, so did your mother when she told you to eat your vegetables, now you are hearing it from us.

Vegetables are full of nutrients and many have antioxidants that will neutralize free radicals, which are molecules that contribute to you developing diseases or aging.

Antioxidants will also help prevent against Alzheimer's, diabetes, stroke, cancer, and heart disease. Be careful to not overcook these, as that will destroy or lessen their nutritional value. Try adding some of these to your diet:

Squash

Red/yellow/orange/green peppers

Dark leafy greens such as kale and spinach

Onions

Asparagus

Mushrooms – try adding mushrooms instead of meat in your recipes to cut calories and cut down on saturated fat. Studies show that mushrooms are just as filling as meat.

Cucumbers

Zucchini

Salad greens

Broccoli

Tomatoes

Yams/sweet potatoes

These foods are low-glycemic foods that will release slowly into your system, and will not cause blood sugar levels to spike.

Not only are these full of antioxidants, but they are low calorie and very filling, making them an excellent side dish to some of your lean proteins for a meal.

Fruits and berries

These are also rich in antioxidants and should be a big part of your diet.

The brighter the color, the more antioxidants they provide.

Most fruits and berries are naturally sweet, but we do not register them as being sweet, because we are so used to the artificially sweetened foods, once you drop the fake sugars from your diet, you will realize how sweet fruits and berries really are.

When feeling your sweet tooth kick in, or just need a pick me up, fruit is the best way to go.

For a nice satisfying sweet tooth fix, a small slice of angel food cake with fresh berries, or some Greek yogurt with either fruit or berries mixed in.

Sprinkle some on your oatmeal if you like, to give it some extra flavor. Suggestions are:

Apples

Grapefruit – a very good food for weight loss, eating half a grapefruit before a meal actually helps you lose weight faster than those who do not.

Blueberries

Bananas

Grapes

Peaches

Pears

Cantaloupe

Strawberries

Oranges

Pineapple

Condiments and sauces

Replace your normal salad dressing, condiments, and sauces with these healthier options.

Fresh salsa or pico de gallo

Guacamole - Avocados contain an unsaturated fat that boosts production of a hormone called lepton, which tells your brain that you are full, so you stop eating

Pesto

Tomato pasta sauce

Curry sauce

Balsamic vinegar

Raspberry vinegar

White cooking wine and red wine.

Raw nuts – almonds, walnuts and pistachios

Nuts are a good protein source and they tend to release their calories slowly, which means that you will feel fuller by eating less.

When you feel the craving to munch, reach for a handful of these nuts instead, along with a glass of water.

Supplements – Do They Work?

No matter what store you go into, in addition to vitamins and minerals you will find all sorts of slimming pills, or fat burning pills, all promising to help you shed pounds just by taking a pill.

Be aware that no pill will ever make you get into shape, with just a pill alone.

Many of these are diuretics, which help you lose water weight.

Others will block, or inhibit the body's ability to digest fat, and can have unpleasant side effects.

There are some things out there that you can take, safely, that will help you reach your weight loss goals however.

Teas – green tea, oolong tea, white tea, and chamomile

Chamomile is a caffeine free tea, and is also very relaxing and can help soothe digestive problems.

Not only that, but it is rich in antioxidants which helps rid your body of stored toxins.

Green tea/oolong tea/white tea/chamomile – All of these are full of antioxidants, phyto chemical and polyphenols, which all help support your immune system and will help you burn off fat quicker.

Green tea also helps reduce belly fat, lowers blood pressure and can help you keep the fat off, once you lose it.

Remember, if you need to sweeten your tea, use Stevia; it is a natural sweetener. You can also use organic honey, as long as it is pure.

If you do not like drinking tea, you can find green tea extracts as a supplement to take in pill form.

Meal replacement bars and shakes

These are designed to be used along with a sensible diet plan and exercise.

The idea is that you replace or two meals (breakfast and/or lunch) with either a meal bar or a shake and then eat a sensible dinner.

These are good, but because they do not have a lot of volume of food, unless you are careful, you might overeat at night, or overdo it on snacks.

We recommend that if you are using these bars and shakes, because they are portable and easy to grab-and-go, that you also have some fruit with it.

Be prepared to have a sensible snack on hand between meals, such as some fruit, raw veggies, nuts, cottage cheese, or yogurt.

Fiber

Anything that will help you feel full is a good thing when dieting, and fiber does just that.

By taking a fiber supplement daily, you will feel fuller after meals and less likely to overeat or snack too much.

You can also increase the fiber that you get by changing your diet to fiber rich foods, but introduce fiber to your system slowly, as too much fiber at one time can make you constipated.

Cayenne pepper

Cayenne and other spicy peppers contain capsaicin, which actually help with appetite suppression. A spicy meal can actually help you to eat less.

Omega-3 fish oil

Omega-3 is not only a natural anti-inflammatory by suppressing cortisol; it also helps increase your body's fat burning capabilities.

The anti-inflammatory nature of this supplement is a good benefit for joint health when exercising.

You can either find these as capsules or you can add more salmon and tuna to your diet.

B Vitamins

By taking a daily B vitamin supplement, you can help ward off the effects of stress, depression and cardiovascular disease as well as promoting healthy skin and muscle tone, enhancing immune system functions and it supports and increases your metabolism.

In addition to a B-Vitamin, you should also take a daily multi-vitamin.

Weight Loss Secrets – Revealed

Okay, so you know what not to eat and you know what to start eating more of, but there must be more to it than just that, right?

Of course there is, and this is the section where we go over all of those weight loss secrets, teaching you not just what to eat, but how to eat to lose weight.

Get plenty of water; you should be drinking between 6-8 glasses of water daily.

Water will help flush out your system, keep your body and skin healthy and best of all, adds no calories.

If you do not like water, add a few slices of orange, lemon, or even lime to your ice water for some extra flavor.

If you are hungry and it is close to mealtime, drink a glass of water to tide you over until mealtime.

The American Diet Association recommends that you have at least 5-9 servings of fruits and vegetables daily.

Start replacing your chips and other calories heavy snacks with snacks that include fruits and vegetables.

Add some to your oatmeal, yogurt or even to cottage cheese. Add then to sandwiches, make them into soups, or use some lean meat to create a stir-fry for some variety.

A very good tip for easy lunches to take to work the next day and for managing your calories when dinning out is to only eat half of the meal and take the other half home to eat as lunch or dinner on a day when you need something fast at hand.

Most restaurant portions are well over what the average person should eat for one meal, and they are usually high in calories, so by turning one meal into two, you get a double benefit there.

Portion control is very important.

Things like ice cream do not need to be totally taken from your diet, but you have to do two things 1) read the labels to make sure that the ice cream is not full of artificial ingredients and 2) see how big a serving size is and stick to it. Yes, invest in a food scale and some measuring cups.

Knowing how much you are eating makes it easier to stick to your calorie count.

Also, invest in a set of small bowls for you to put your snacks in, no more eating from the bag, or just guessing your portion size.

For example, if you want ice cream, measure out ½ of a cup and put it in a small bowl.

If you have a larger bowl, and want ice cream, and you do not measure it, you are very likely to have more than just the suggested serving size of ½.

By using a smaller bowl or even a smaller plate at mealtime, you are not seeing as much empty space, making you think that you are not eating as much as you really are.

Although it seems contrary to dieting, do not deny yourself food or your favorite treat.

If you deny that nagging voice about a craving for very long, by the time you give in, instead of just a small amount, you end up over indulging on it.

Along the same lines of thinking, buy those snack packs of snacks.

If you buy a whole box of cookies, it is easier to eat a bunch of cookies than if you did not have access to a bunch of cookies.

If you buy your snacks in bulk, to avoid overeating, put them in small snack size Ziploc bags or containers and allow yourself to only grab one bag, or container at a time.

Not only does this make it easier for you to grab and go, but it is a great way for portion control and to satisfy cravings without binging.

Have some protein with every meal, protein satisfies better than fats and carbohydrates, and so getting enough protein helps you feel fuller while encouraging fat burning and preserving muscle mass.

You can incorporate cheese, nuts, and yogurt into your snacks to help you feel fuller with less.

Beans are a good source of protein and including them in your meals is a great idea.

Forget out the three meals a day only plan. Eat smaller meals and incorporate snacks into your day to avoid those periods of hunger, which is when you are likely to overeat.

Bring your own lunch to work. Avoid the fast food trap and stop making eating out a daily thing.

Although you can find healthy alternatives when you eat out, it is much easier when you bring your own lunch, that way you can easier track the calorie intake.

A Few Ideas for What to Eat

For a quick easy salad, you can use bagged salad greens with some grilled chicken or turkey breast along with some cheese and vegetables.

Whole-grain wraps and pitas can be combined with any combination of lean meat, salad, cheese, and lettuce for a tasty sandwich wrap.

You can combine black beans, rice and lean meat and cheese for a tasty and low calorie burrito as well.

Make things like black beans and rice ahead of time, and keep them in the fridge so you can very easily assemble a fast meal, or to pack a lunch for you to take to work.

You can even find pre-cooked brown rice in most grocery stores. You can combine just the brown rice with black beans and salsa in a whole-wheat tortilla for a tasty burrito.

Keep canned beans on hand, such as kidney beans, black beans, and lentils.

Canned diced tomatoes are also good to keep on hand for making handy meals.

Combine canned tomatoes with onion and use as a salsa to put over chicken for dinner instead of your normal sauce. It will be fewer calories and still have plenty of flavor.

Microwave popcorn makes a great snack, if you buy the light version. Fast to make and averages about 25 calories per cup.

For a handy supply of pre-cooked chicken breasts, instead of buying the sliced, pre-cooked chicken breasts in the store, which can be loaded with preservatives, buy a pack of chicken breasts and cook them, keep them in the fridge to add to salads, wraps, or to use in your nighttime meals.

Yogurt, cheese, and cottage cheese are all versatile foods, which can be mixed and matched with fruits and vegetables for snacks or a light meal. Try a pear, a yogurt and one piece of string cheese.

Canned tuna and salmon can be combined with a small about of fat free mayonnaise or better yet, Dijon mustard with some diced onion.

Wrap up in a whole-wheat wrap or tortilla along with whatever vegetables you would like to add, such as lettuce, peppers, or tomatoes for example.

Need a snack but just a piece of fruit is not satisfying enough?

Cut an apple into wedges eat with some natural peanut butter, or use the apple wedges to scoop up some cottage cheese or yogurt.

Top a baked potato with salsa, low fat cottage cheese, or low fat cheddar cheese.

Use frozen vegetables and a variety of vegetables to cook a stir-fry, using olive oil to cook with and pair with brown rice.

Make hard-boiled eggs ahead of time and mix with Dijon mustard and tuna or salmon to either put in a wrap or to be eaten over salad greens.

Add a hard-boiled egg to your salads, or just as a side item to go with your lunch.

Pair a chicken breast with brown rice and steamed broccoli or other vegetables – if you have already cooked chicken breast and rice at home, you will have a simple meal with very little preparation required.

Mix cottage cheese with any combination of fruit that you would like and eat with one serving of whole-wheat crackers – this makes a great lunch.

Try hummus on a whole-wheat pita for a snack, or add salad greens and make into a wrap for light meal.

Use canned tomatoes and beans to make chili with ground turkey.

Tomatoes and cucumbers, with some non-fat mozzarella, drizzled with olive oil and balsamic vinegar on pita bread makes for a nice lunch.

No Excuses

Okay, the easy part is over with, the diet part. Now we are going to focus on the second and equally important part, the exercise plan.

To get into shape, you need to incorporate exercises as well as diet changes.

Everybody want to get into shape, but nobody wants to do the work, or they say they do, but they have a whole arsenal of excuses as to why they want to exercise but cannot.

We are about to list those common excuses and shoot them all down.

There is no excuse to not starting to get healthy.

Exercise is monotonous

Yes, it can be, but it does not have to be monotonous.

Break up your exercise routine so you are not doing the same old thing every time.

Take up a sport that will not be boring, we guarantee that!

You can also take a fitness class or even a sports class at the local community center.

Turn exercise time into family time and go for a bike ride with the whole family.

Do a mixture of strength and cardio to avoid the same old routine.

If you are using home fitness equipment, thwart boredom by watching TV or situate your computer or laptop where you can see it and play movies.

This keeps you from focusing on just the monotony of the equipment, and your time will go by faster.

It is overwhelming

Yes, when you are overweight, it can be overwhelming to get into shape, but that is why we went over setting goals first.

Because, when you set a bunch of smaller goals, it does not look so overwhelming and you will not be as stressed out about your workout and diet plan.

Afraid to fail

So many people are afraid to set and follow their goals because they are afraid that they will not be able to commit and that they will fail.

All we have to say is this, if you do not try, you will never have the chance to succeed or fail.

This is why we have set you up to replace your junk food with better food slowly, and to set your smaller goals for your weight loss, exercise, and lifestyle changes.

We understand how hard it is when you change everything suddenly, so have you gradually making the changes, no big commitment to change all at once.

I am afraid it will hurt

We will not kid you, you will feel sore and you will have aches and pains, but nothing compared to the damage that being overweight does to your body.

If you get injured, or feel more than just muscle soreness from using muscles you are not used to doing, stop!

Never push yourself into the zone where you are hurt, no exercise plan should ever require you of that.

Small goals, we are easing you into this, never just go all in to a major exercise plan.

I do not have enough time

Actually, you do. You can get into shape without spending a ton of time on it, you just need to set aside some time daily, and you would be surprised how you can fit getting fit into your day.

Cardio

Cardio exercises are the best way to burn fat, lose weight, and keep it off, and it helps strengthen your heart, lowering your risk of developing heart disease.

For cardio to be effective, you must get into your target heart rate zone, a casual stroll at a leisurely pace, never breaking a sweat will not have any benefits in terms of cardio.

It will help you burn calories, so any walking is good, but it does not count as cardio.

We are going to be suggesting that you follow a progressive pattern for cardio, so we will start slow and then increase the pace, the length, and the number of days per week that you will be exercising.

How do you know what your target heart rate is? Your maximum heart rate is 220 beats per minute – your age.

Your target heart rate is between 50-85% of your maximum heart rate.

We are suggesting that for the beginning stages of your workouts, which you go for 50%, so that you do not overdo it.

Therefore you take 220 and subtract your age and multiply by 50% to find your target heart rate.

Once you are more used to doing cardio, you can up it to 55%, then 58%, up to a maximum of 85%.

To take your pulse you will need a clock or a watch with either a stopwatch function or a second hand.

With your first two fingers over your pulse, count the number of beats you feel in a 10 second period and multiply by 6. That is your beats per minute.

Alternatively, you can measure it more simply, if you can still carry on a conversation with ease, then you are not at your target heart rate zone.

If it costs you a little to moderate effort, you are in the low to low-middle range of your target heart rate.

If you have trouble talking while doing your cardio or it requires a lot of effort you are in the medium to medium-high target heart rate, and if you are only able to carry on a conversation by exerting maximum effort or if you are unable to speak, you are in the high ranges of your target heart rate, and should dial back the intensity a notch or two.

Before, during and after your cardio you will need to drink plenty of water.

Keeping hydrated is very important.

What types of exercises count as being cardio?

Here are some examples:

Walking/jogging/running

Jumping

Swimming

Rowing

Bicycling

Aerobics

Stair climbing

Roller skating

Those are just a few examples; there are really endless possibilities for cardio of all levels.

Anything that gets your heartbeat above normal will count as cardio.

Cardio can be broken down into intensity and duration and here are some main ways to combine those into effective workouts:

Low Intensity workouts with a long duration

Workouts in this category are designed to keep your target heart rate between 40%-60% of your maximum heart rate

Workouts in this category are designed to be 40 minutes or longer in duration

You should be able to carry on a conversation comfortably while working out

Excellent for people just starting to get into shape

Excellent way to lose weight

Medium Intensity workouts with a medium duration

Workouts in this category are designed to keep your target heart rate at about 70% of your maximum heart rate.

Workouts in this category are designed to be between 20-30 minutes in duration

You should have difficulty carrying on a conversation while working out

Excellent for weight loss, and increasing your cardiovascular endurance

High Intensity workouts with a short duration

Workouts in this category are designed to keep your target heart rate between 80-85% of your maximum heart rate

Workouts in this category are designed to only 5-20 minutes in duration

Extremely demanding and you should not be able to carry on a conversation

Your target heart rate should never exceed 85%

For experienced people only, this should only be for those who are already physically fit, not designed for those getting into shape

Interval Training

Alternating between medium to high intensity exercise and low intensity exercise

Example – run 5 minutes at 60% of your maximum heart rate, followed by 2 minutes of slow walking, and then another 5 minutes of running at 60% of your maximum heart beat again

Flexible way to tailor your workout to your fitness level

Works best when you vary the intensity but do not stop completely in between

Best results for weight loss

Beginning Your Workout

Okay, so now that you understand what cardio is, now we can go over how to begin your cardio workouts.

Remember, if you are not used to exercising, or are very out of shape, the goal is to just get moving and stay in motion for about 20 minutes, about three days a week.

Worry about moderate and interval workouts only after you have built up your endurance.

Increase your workout time by 5 minutes each week. You may think that 5 minutes every week is not a big deal, but trust us, it will be.

To begin with, make sure you have comfortable shoes and a good pair of socks. It sounds basic, but being able to exercise without getting blisters is a necessity.

Make sure that if you are going to be running, that you have running shoes, if you are going to be doing low impact type cardio, you can use cross-trainers or running shoes.

Most sports have a specific shoe designed for that sport, so always get the appropriate shoe.

Your clothing should be comfortable, and not too loose, you do not want it to get caught in any machines, or trip over pants that are too long.

For example, yoga requires clothing that is not loose, so you can move freely and jogging requires nothing more than shorts and a t-shirt.

Always start-off with stretching and a few minutes of warm up.

Your warm up session should last about 5-10 minutes at a light intensity.

Warming up helps to prevent injuries or strains and prepares your body for the upcoming workout.

Pick a cardio activity that you like. You can choose to use equipment such as a stationary bike, treadmill, stair stepper or elliptical.

You can even take a class or buy a DVD for aerobics, step, Zumba, or any other class type cardio work out.

For beginners, always start with beginning classes, you can try yoga, either in a class or at home, or you can invest in a stability ball, which will combine cardio with some core training.

You can also walk around your neighborhood, a park, etc., or jog or run, ride a bike, swim or even take up a sport.

Pick an activity that sounds interesting to you and one that you would enjoy doing, because you will be challenging yourself.

As you begin to exercise, you should pay attention to your breathing.

Breathe in through your nose, out through your mouth, and slow down if you start having trouble breathing.

As your cardiovascular system improves, your breathing will no longer be as labored, this means that you are doing something right.

Check your target heart range often, especially when you are first getting started with your fitness regimen, you should be in your target heart rate range for at least 20 minutes for your work out to be effective, as you build up endurance, you extend the duration of your work out by 5 minutes every week.

After you are comfortable with your intensity and duration, you up your intensity to a slightly higher target heart rate, and then start off slow again, working back up to longer duration by 5 minutes a week.

Always have a cool down period.

Gradually slow your speed down let your heart rate come down, and do this for about 5 minutes, gradually slowing down and then stop. Finish up by a stretching session.

Feel free to change up your routine, add new elements, or switch your elements around, especially if you are using interval training.

We suggest that you wait until you can comfortably do moderate intensity exercises before starting interval training, to avoid pushing your body too far.

Strength Training

On the days that you are not doing cardio, you can do your strength training.

We realize that not everybody has access to a gym, where you have a ton of equipment, so we will try to focus mostly on the exercises that you can do at home.

We do recommend that you invest in a set of hand weights, a resistance band, or even a stability ball. Stability balls combine cardio with core training and strength training.

Do your strength training anywhere from 1-3 days a week, on the days that you do not do cardio.

Always give yourself a day of rest in between strength training sessions.

Do not overdo it, for the first month or two; just concentrate on learning the exercises and how to do them properly, not on how many you can do, or how much weight you can lift.

You will impress nobody if you hurt yourself by trying to take on too much at once.

Every week, add another repetition to each exercise, or if you are using weights, add another pound.

You should be starting with 1 or 2 sets of 10-16 repetitions of each exercise.

We suggest starting with only 1 set for the first few weeks, to give your body time to adjust and to get used to the workout.

After the first month, add a second set.

Once you have built your strength up, then you can add more reps, but never go above 16 reps per set.

If using weights, each time you add weight, drop your reps down; so if you are using 5 pound weights, and doing 1 set of 16 reps at 5 pounds, when you go to 6 pounds, you do 1 set of 12 reps, until you are comfortable with the weight, then you can increase your reps back up slowly to 16.

How do you know how many sets and reps to do?

See below:

If your goal is to lose body fat and build muscle

Use enough weight so that you can only comfortably complete 10-12 repetitions

1 set for beginners, 2 for intermediate and advanced exercisers should do three

Rest 30 seconds to 1 minute between sets

If your goal is to gain muscle

Use enough weight so that you can only complete comfortably 4-8 reps

3 or more sets with 1-2 minutes in-between

Not for beginners to strength training

2-3 days in between each session

To keep in shape

Use enough weight so that you can only comfortably complete 12-16 reps

1-3 sets depending on your endurance and comfort

Resting 20-30 seconds between sets

If you do not have dumbbells, you can always make your own weights to use at home; here are some ideas:

Buckets – fill some small (or large) buckets with as much water or sand as you want – you can easily adjust your weight by taking out or adding sand or water.

Hold the buckets by the handle when doing your exercises.

This is good to use with step-ups and squats, lunges, etc., just nothing that requires you to lift this over your head or tip it.

Milk bottles – using gallon or half-gallon milk bottles are a good way to make your own weights, because these have handle for you to grip onto when using them.

This is a great option for bicep curls, bent-over rows and tricep extensions, lunges, etc.

Here are some easy to do strength training exercises that you can do at home, without buying extra equipment.

Pushups

Easy to do, using your own body weight to strengthen your muscles; this is the most common strength training exercise.

To start, place your palms flat on the ground, directly under your shoulders, and have your toes on the ground, keeping your back straight.

Tighten your abs and push yourself up, until your arms are full extended, then lower yourself back towards the ground, but not all the way, then back up.

You can turn this into an advanced exercise by placing your feet on stop of step, a bed, or even a chair.

Leg Raises

Excellent for working your lower abs.

Lay flat on your back with your arms at your sides and lift your legs straight up into the air, until your heels are parallel to the ceiling, then lower your legs back to the floor.

If you feel discomfort in your back when doing this, place both hands behind your back, flat on the floor, under your tailbone.

To make this more advanced, alternate lifting and lowering your legs separately, like a pair of scissors, when one goes up, the other goes down.

Lunges

Lunges are excellent for working quads, hamstrings, calves, and glutes.

Start off standing with your feet together and then take one giant step forward.

Lower yourself until your front knee is at a 90-degree angle and your back knee should be just above the ground.

Now lift your back foot, and take another giant step forward, until your front knee is at a 90-degree angle and your back knee is just above the ground.

Your front knee should never be past your ankle and your back should always be straight. Go as far across the room this way as you can, then turn around and repeat.

Dips

Dips will work the triceps. You will need two chairs, spread your legs apart and put a chair by each foot.

Stand between the two chairs, placing your hands on the edge of one chair and your heels on the edge of the other chair and slowly lower your body down until your arms are bent at 90 degrees, and then push yourself back up.

Burpees

These are both cardio and strength training, and should be done fast, in as smooth as a motion as you can.

Stand straight with your arms by your sides, feet hip width apart, drop to a squat.

Now kick your legs out behind you, extend your arms and do a pushup, as you rise up from the pushup, go back to the squat position, jump up in the air, come back to the squat position.

Sit-ups

Another classic exercise, great for losing belly fat and building abs.

Lay down flat on the floor.

Bend your knees, the degree of the bend will be up to you, only you know how comfortable you will be when doing this. Experiment some with this.

Your feet should be on the ground; you can even have somebody holding your feet, or stick your feet under a chair or bed to help to avoid raising your feet off of the ground.

Place your hands on the side of your head, or clasp them behind your neck, but do not push on your head or neck when doing the exercise!

Your elbows should now be pointed outwards, towards your knees.

Raise your upper body towards your knees, going slowly, until you touch your elbow to your knees, hold the position for two seconds, and then slowly lower yourself back to the floor.

Squats

Squats will help strengthen calves, glutes, and quads.

Stand upright, with your feet shoulder length apart, bend at the knees, until your thighs are parallel to the floor, slowly raise back to the standing position.

Superman/superwoman

No, this will not make your faster than a speeding bullet, but it will work your upper, middle, and lower back all at once.

Get down to all fours on the floor. Your back and neck should be straight.

Raise up your left arm in front of you while lifting your right leg up behind you until they are both straight, so your body is in line.

Hold this for 30 seconds then repeat with your right arm and left leg.

Plank pose

This is like a pushup, only without the push.

You get into the pushup positions, hands extended under your body and toes on the ground, holding your body straight, your head and neck in line with your spine.

Hold the pose for as long as you can.

Reverse crunches

Lie on the floor, on your back, lay your arms flat out to your sides, and then raise your legs into the air, lifting your hips off of the ground.

To make this an advanced exercise, cross your arms over your chest.

Leg curls

Start off on all fours, but instead of having your hands flat on the ground, lean forward so that your forearms are on the ground and your knees are under your hips.

Extend one leg behind you, then bend it at the knee, straighten and repeat. Switch legs.

Bent over row

Start of standing next to a sturdy and stable surface, such as a bed or a coffee table.

If using a coffee table, put a folded towel down to cushion the surface.

Place your right hand and right knee on the surface, hold either a dumbbell or a homemade weight in your left hand and slowly bring it up to the side of your chest, keeping your back straight.

Lower the weight until the arm holding the weight is straight again. Repeat and then switch sides.

Step-ups

Using a stair or low stool or ledge, stand just in front of the step; feet shoulder length apart and your arms down by your side or on your hips.

Step up onto the step with one leg first, pause when both feet are on the step.

Step down with the foot that was opposite of the one you started to step with, then the other foot. Switch which foot you lead with; repeat.

You can do this holding weights if you like.

Wall squat

Stand slightly away from a wall, and then lean back into the wall.

Your feet should be about two feet away from the wall, shoulder width apart and flat on the ground.

Bend your knees to lower yourself slightly down the wall and hold it for 10 seconds.

Bend your knees even more and then hold for 10 seconds again, continue slowly going down the wall, pausing for 10 seconds each time, until you cannot go any lower.

Lateral Raises

This requires you to use either dumbbells or homemade weights, which we went over above. Stand with your feet shoulder width apart, with a weight in each hand, down at your sides.

Raise both arms at the same time, until they are even with your shoulders, keeping your elbows just slightly bent.

Do not jerk the weights; use a fluid motion to raise your arms.

Conclusion

We have given you the tools, now it is up to you to put it all together.

By following our simple food guidelines and our progressive exercises, you will be able to get into shape quickly and to stay that way.

You need to switch your thinking that dieting is about taking away from what you eat.

It is less about what you do not eat and more about what you add into your diet, or replace your diet with.

No diet should ever require you to feel hungry, or to starve yourself, so we have come up with a plan that allows you to still eat, but to do it sensibly, and in a healthy way.

The goal to dieting is not just to lose weight, but to be healthier, which is why fad diets just do not work. They are a short-term fix only.

Our method of slowly phasing out the foods that you should not eat, and adding in the foods that you should is a great way to not only start your path to being healthy and losing weight, but by keeping it off.

This is not crash diet, it is a lifestyle change that will have you looking and feeling better in no time at all.

Along with our easy diet guidelines, we have also gone over how to incorporate both cardio and strength training into your routine, to help you lose weight and build muscle faster than dieting alone.

Our progressive plan starts you off slow and easy, letting you set the pace, and your comfort zone. Only you can tell how much is too much, and how fast is too fast.

Remember to monitor your target heart rate, and never let it get above 85% of your maximum heart rate.

You will not lose weight faster by pushing yourself; you will only cause harm.

Pick and choose between the suggested exercises, but by all means, you are not limited to what we have listed.

Classes are a great way to meet other people with the same goals as you, and can put a fun and different spin on your routine.

You can also find any number of DVDS's to use at home as well. For beginners, yoga is a great way to increase your flexibility and learn to breathe properly while exercising; it is a great way to shed stress as well.

You know when you are ready to move your routine up to the next level, add a few more minutes of cardio, and add a few more reps or another pound of weight.

Keep challenging yourself, while eating healthy and see the new you come through.

www.ingramcontent.com/pod-product-compliance
Lightning Source LLC
Chambersburg PA
CBHW020356290526
45785CB00005B/2307